How To Stop Snoring Forever

334 Great Tips To Get Rid Of Snoring

ADAM COLTON

Published by BizMove
www.bizmove.com

ISBN: 1978475861
ISBN- 978-1978475861

Table of Contents

1. Snoring Fact Sheet

Snoring is a loud, hoarse, harsh breathing sound that occurs during sleep. Snoring is common in adults.

Loud, frequent snoring can make it hard for both you and your bed partner to get enough sleep. Sometimes snoring can be a sign of a sleep disorder called sleep apnea.

Causes

When you sleep, the muscles in your throat relax and your tongue slips back in your mouth. Snoring occurs when something blocks air from flowing freely through your mouth and nose. When you breathe, the walls of your throat vibrate, causing the sound of snoring.

There are several factors that can lead to snoring, including

- Being overweight. The extra tissue in your neck puts pressure on your airways.
- Tissue swelling during the last month of pregnancy.

- Crooked or bent nasal septum, which is the wall of bone and cartilage between your nostrils.
- Growths in your nasal passages (nasal polyps).
- Stuffy nose from a cold or allergies.
- Swelling in the roof of your mouth (soft palate) or the uvula, the piece of tissue that hangs down in the back of your mouth. These areas may also be longer than normal.
- Swollen adenoids and tonsils that block the airways. This is a common cause of snoring in children.
- A tongue that is wider at the base, or a larger tongue in a smaller mouth.
- Poor muscle tone. This may be caused by aging or by using sleeping pills, antihistamines, or alcohol at bedtime.

Sometimes snoring can be a sign of a sleep disorder called sleep apnea.

- This occurs when you completely or partly stop breathing for more than 10 seconds while you sleep.
- This is followed by a sudden snort or gasp when you start breathing again. During that time you wake up without realizing it.
- Then you start to snore again.
- This cycle usually happens many times a night, which makes it hard to sleep deeply.

Sleep apnea can make it especially hard for your bed partner to get a good night's sleep.

Home Care

To help reduce snoring:

- Avoid alcohol and medicines that make you sleepy at bedtime.
- DO NOT sleep flat on your back. Try to sleep on your side instead. You can sew a golf or tennis ball into the back of your night clothes. If you roll over, the pressure of the ball will help remind you to stay on your side. Over time, side sleeping will become a habit.
- Lose weight, if you are overweight.
- Try over-the-counter, drug-free nasal strips that help widen the nostrils. (These are not treatments for sleep apnea.)

If your health care provider has given you a breathing device, use it on a regular basis. Follow your provider's advice for treating allergy symptoms.

When to Call Your Doctor

Talk to your health care provider if you:

- Have problems with attention, concentration, or memory

- Wake up in the morning not feeling rested
- Feel very drowsy during the day
- Have morning headaches
- Gain weight
- Tried self-care for snoring, and it has not helped

You should also talk with your provider if you have episodes of no breathing (apnea) during the night. Your partner can tell you if you are snoring loudly or making choking and gasping sounds.

Depending on your symptoms and the cause of your snoring, your provider may refer you to a sleep specialist.

2. 334 Great Tips To Get Rid Of Snoring

Many people are affected by snoring. Perhaps you tend to snore, or maybe you wish your spouse would sleep more quietly. Snoring can affect relationships in negative ways. Regardless of whether it is you or a loved one who snores, the following advice will help.

1. Sleep more upright. Elevating your upper body can relieve both gravity and pressure, allowing you to get a full night's rest without snoring. Use pillows or put some bricks under the headboard. Even just a slight elevation can stop you from snoring, so try it out and see what height works best for you.

2. Stick to a regular bedtime, and practice good sleep habits in general to reduce the incidence of snoring. If you go to bed overtired, sleep erratic hours, or have other bad sleep habits, you may sleep very deeply which relaxes the muscles in the back of your throat more than usual. This can contribute to snoring.

3. When you are pregnant, you should talk to your doctor. immediately. if you snore constantly.

Although many expectant mothers do snore during pregnancy because of the extra pressure on their bodies, it is important to make sure that your baby still has enough oxygen while you are snoring. Ask your doctor for advice on how to prevent problems that snoring can cause your baby.

4. Excessive snoring can sometimes keep you from getting a restful night's sleep, but if you do snore never take sleeping pills. Sleeping pills cause every muscle in your body to relax, including the muscles in your jaw and neck. This will only serve to make your snoring problems worse and severe problems like sleep apnea can develop.

5. To keep yourself from snoring, eat your largest meal of the day at least a few hours before bed. If you hop into bed with a full stomach, it will apply pressure to your diaphragm, pushing it up and narrowing your air passageways -- and making you snore. Eat earlier so you can digest your food -- and not snore.

6. To help alleviate snoring, try to use over-the-counter snoring aids that help to open your airway. Snoring is often caused by the airway being constricted. By simply changing how you breathe, snoring can be relieved. There are many products

available that can help open your airway, without needing to take any pills.

7. In order to reduce snoring you should not drink alcohol or take any kind of sedative or relaxant, including antihistamines for several hours before bedtime. Any of these things make the muscles in your body relax. Relaxed muscles close up your airway even further than normal. The blockage can cause snoring or make it worse than usual.

8. Make sure that you find a comfortable position when lying down to sleep. One of the reasons that you will snore during the night is because of a lack of comfort when you lay down. Reduce the strain on your body to limit snoring in an effort to optimize the coziness of your night.

9. Start an exercise program. Snoring can be caused by not being in good shape. As you exercise and the muscles in your arms and legs become stronger and more toned, so will your throat muscles. Well-developed and toned throat muscles decrease the chance of your snoring because your throat remains open.

10. Eating smaller evening meals can reduce snoring. A larger meal close to bedtime will fill up the stomach. This pushes up the diaphragm and can

block up your throat. Reduced air flow and a narrow throat are two of the main factors in snoring.

11.   If your snoring stops intermittently during the night, and you wake up gasping for a breath, you should make an appointment to see your doctor. This is because you may have sleep apnea, which is a serious disorder. If someone tells you that this is your sleep pattern, a sleep study may need to be conducted on you to confirm this condition.

12.   Take a good hot shower before going to bed. Not only will it relax you and help you get to sleep, the steam from the shower will moisturize and open your respiratory passages. When you are dry inside you are more likely to snore. The steam will remedy that problem.

13.   Losing weight is a good step to take in order to stop snoring at night while you are asleep. Extra weight restricts breathing, especially extra weight around the neck. Maintain a balanced diet, exercise, and lose a few pounds to help remedy your breathing and snoring issues.

14.   Allergies can cause snoring because they make people breathe through their mouths while sleeping. If you have bad allergies, an antihistamine works

great, as does other nasal sprays. If your nose is stopped up, there is a good chance you will be snoring at night. Clear your breathing passages in efforts to stop snoring.

15.   Talk to your doctor about the advisability of being fitted for a mandibular advancement appliance. You will need to have an appliance like this fitted into your mouth, resting against your teeth. The appliance positions your jaw slightly forward, which can help you stop snoring.

16.   One of the oldest methods to prevent snoring is the use of a chin strap. Their design has changed over the years so that the new ones are quite comfortable. They keep your mouth from opening at night so that are not breathing through your mouth. Thus, you must breathe through your nose, which keeps you from snoring.

17.   One simple exercise that you can do to help prevent snoring is to say your vowels. Take a few minutes a few times a day to say a, e, i, o and u. Say each letter loudly and draw out the sound to last 5-10 seconds each. This will help strengthen throat muscles that are lax and eliminate snoring.

18.   If you regularly use cigarettes and other tobacco products, you probably also snore. The ingredients

in these products dries out the mucosal membranes in your nose, mouth and airway, which leads to difficulty breathing and loud snoring. If at all possible, do not smoke cigarettes within five hours of your bedtime as the smoke will cause your airway to become inflamed.

19.   Try not to take any medications that contain sedatives, if you want to stop snoring. Sedatives are known to relax the throat muscles and when these muscles are too relaxed, snoring occurs. If you medications have sedatives, speak with your doctor about switching to a similar medication that does not have a sedative.

20.   If you are over weight, snoring might be a problem. To make that problem stop, lose the excess pounds. Extra weight is stored in many different areas on your body, including in your neck. The fat stored in your neck region causes the throat to constrict, which often results in snoring. When you take off those extra pounds, the snoring will often come to an end.

21.   Avoid alcoholic beverages and sleep-inducing pills like tranquilizers or antihistamines close to bedtime. When muscles are relaxed by these artificial properties, they tend to get restrict your air passages. This restriction will increase snoring and

keep you up. If you're going to drink alcohol, do it earlier in the evening.

22.   If you suffer from chronic snoring, you may benefit from allergy testing. Allergies can clog the nasal passages and force you to breathe out of your mouth, which causes snoring. Finding out the causes of your allergies allows you to eliminate their sources. Also, you may benefit from taking a prescribed or over-the-counter antihistamine before bed.

23.   Try to to avoid consuming alcohol right before bed. Alcohol does help you relax; the problem is drinking alcohol right before bed causes the muscles of your airway to relax too much. This over relaxation causes snoring which you may not notice. but, people around you will definitely be disturbed.

24.   Blow your nose well before you go to bed. Often snoring is caused by a buildup of mucous in your nose. A stopped-up nose typically causes you to open your mouth during your sleep in order to breathe. When you breathe through your mouth you snore so keep some tissue at the side of your bed to prevent the problem before it starts.

25.   You may want to think about getting a mouth device to prevent breathing through your mouth

when you sleep. Breathing through your mouth, and not your nose, can cause snoring. These mouth devices block breathing through your mouth and encourage you to breathe through your nose instead. Speak with your doctor about this option.

26.   In order to stop snoring, go to your local pharmacy and buy some nasal strips. You don't have to put them on until bedtime. The benefit is that the strips will make your nasal passageways open up and permit more air flow. The end result is that you will snore much less.

27.   To limit your level of snoring during the night, refrain from smoking altogether. Smoking can constrict your airways, which can make it much harder for you to breathe at night. This will not only help you to reduce the intensity of your snoring but make you feel better as the night wears on.

28.   If you want to stop snoring, talk to your dentist or physician about a mouth guard. The purpose of the guard is to keep your teeth together, and to ensure that the lower jaw muscles do not relax so much that your air passageways slacken, and snoring starts again. That's the last thing you want!

29.   Ready to stop snoring? There are some throat exercises you can do to keep your throat muscles

stronger. One thing you can do is repeat the five vowels out loud, consistently, for three minutes consecutively, several times a day. Building your throat muscles will reduce your instances of snoring.

30.   Smoking tobacco makes snoring worse, so people that snore should quit smoking. Until you can quit, you should limit your smoking as much as possible, especially before bedtime. Smoking causes your throat, mouth, and nasal passages to swell up and become inflamed. If you do not smoke for several hours before bed, your tissues have a chance of returning to normal which will help reduce your snoring.

31.   Lose as much excess weight as possible. Extra weight does not just show up in your thighs, it can make your throat narrower. This can cause snoring and sleep apnea. Even a 10 pound loss can help open up the passageway in your throat. The more wide open it is, the better you will sleep.

32.   Make an effort to sing every day, as much as you can. People have noticed that the more they sing, the less they snore. Singing helps develop and strengthen the throat and mouth muscles. The stronger your throat muscles are, the less you snore.

Strong throat muscles are less likely to collapse or become blocked.

33.   Purchase nasal strips that help keep your nasal passages open at night. The strips are applied to your skin across the bridge of your nose. If you can breathe easily through your nose, then you will probably keep your mouth shut at night. Breathing through an open mouth is one of the biggest causes of snoring.

34.   Smoking causes your throat to swell, which in turn causes you to snore at night. One good way to prevent snoring is to stop smoking now. Try a smoking cessation class, over-the-counter nicotine patches or a prescription medication from your doctor. You will not only improve your health and prevent lung cancer, but you will sleep better at night.

35.   In order to cut back on snoring, turn over and sleep on your side, not on your back. If you sleep on your back, especially with only one or two pillows, mucus can gather in your nasal passages. Sleeping on your side will keep the mucus out of the passages, and you won't have a blockage that will cause snoring.

36.   Consider using a chin strap to keep your snoring under control. Chin straps keep your mouth closed so it is difficult to snore. These devices are available in a wide variety of styles. Many are elastic and simply fit over your head. Others are fitted with Velcro so they can be custom adjusted to fit your head.

37.   Avoid snoring by staying away from food that is high in carbs, especially late in the day. Foods like pizza, cake, and cookies can fill up your stomach and cause it to push on your diaphragm. This will squeeze your air passages, making it harder for air to get through -- and causing you to snore.

38.   You may want to look into magnetic therapy in order to end snoring. With this method, a plastic ring with two magnetic ends attach to your nose when you go to sleep. The ring helps to stimulate the sensors that open the nasal passages, thus, preventing a person from snoring.

39.   Sleep on your side to minimize your chances of snoring. If you sleep on your back, your tongue may fall back into your throat and obstruct the airways. This can result in snoring. Sleeping on your side keeps the tongue from falling back into the throat, so you are less likely to snore.

40.   Practice good sleep hygiene to combat snoring. Sleep hygiene refers to developing good sleep habits, such as sleeping at the same time each day and getting enough sleep each night. Try to maintain the same sleep schedule 7 days a week, whether you are working or not. Also, make sure you get at least 7 or 8 hours of sleep every night.

41.   Try to not consume overly sugary foods or overly rich foods. Deserts, in particular, aren't a good choice when you have a tendency to snore. Chocolates, cookies, cakes, and even ice cream are associated with snoring. So too are foods such a pizza, lasagna, and other high-calorie, high-fat, rich foods.

42.   A tennis ball might be a simple solution to your snoring problems. Pin this ball to your nightwear before bed. While you are sleeping, you will naturally turn on your side when you feel the tennis ball on your back. Sleeping to the side is an effective way to reduce the snoring.

43.   If all of your remedies fail, one of the things that you can do is seek professional advice from a doctor. There are many different types of surgeries that you can undergo to increase your air passages so that you can breathe more efficiently at night.

Get professional help if your snoring becomes a serious dilemma.

44.   Avoid sleeping on your back to reduce nightly snoring. If you can not avoid sleeping on your back, you should try to attach a large- sized item to the back side of your pajamas. This will cause you to be uncomfortable if you roll onto your back while sleeping, and you will quickly re-position.

45.   To minimize snoring, try to eat a large breakfast and lunch during the day. This will force you to have a smaller dinner, which is very beneficial towards maintaining a high comfort level when you sleep at night. The more comfortable you are when you rest, the less of a chance for you to snore.

46.   To reduce snoring, train yourself to breathe through your nose. There are snoring strips on the market that adhere across the bridge of the nose. They open the nasal passages to encourage nasal breathing. These can be used in conjunction with chin straps to prevent the mouth from opening while you sleep.

47.   Do you snore? Give singing a try. Singing is a natural form of exercise for the muscles in the throat and soft palate. Since snoring is sometimes caused by lax muscles in these areas, strengthening

them can help. So go ahead and belt out your favorite tune every day. Your partner might just sleep better because they no longer have to listen to you snore!

48. If you are pregnant and snoring often, you need to see your doctor. Sometimes the extra pounds along with certain hormonal changes cause pregnant women to snore more often. This deprives the baby of oxygen, so this is an issue that needs to be addressed right away by paying a visit to your doctor.

49. If you are becoming a nuisance to yourself and someone you love because of snoring, try this tip. Oils, such as peppermint, eucalyptus and menthol have been known to shrink nasal passages, reducing the chances of snoring. Just rub a little around your nostril opening and you should notice a decrease in your snoring.

50. There are some hereditary abnormalities that a person can be born with that increases the likelihood of him or her snoring at night. Also, men have a narrow nasal passageway compared to women, increasing their chances of snoring more than women. Learn what you can do in order to prevent snoring according to your unique situation.

51.   To help stop snoring problems, try to avoid taking sleeping pills or other types of tranquilizing medication to help you rest. These sleep aids may help you feel more restful, but they also contribute to both snoring and sleep apnea. Some tranquilizers are even addictive and can cause health problems if overused.

52.   Avoid drinking alcohol within 5 hours of bedtime. Alcohol, along with other sedative drugs, causes the muscles at the back of the throat to relax. When these muscles relax, you are more apt to snore. Stay away from those nightcaps--you may actually sleep more soundly if you do not drink before bed.

53.   If you often find yourself snoring at night, avoid drinking alcohol. Alcohol can suppress the central nervous system, thus causing all the muscles in your throat to fall into a relaxed state. Your jaw muscles will relax too, increasing any snoring problems. Only drink in moderation, if at all, and you will avoid this problem.

54.   If you suffer from chronic snoring, you may benefit from allergy testing. Allergies can clog the nasal passages and force you to breathe out of your mouth, which causes snoring. Finding out the causes of your allergies allows you to eliminate their

sources. Also, you may benefit from taking a prescribed or over-the-counter antihistamine before bed.

55.   Tape your nose using specialized strips. Snoring is not only a problem in regard to your health, it can impact the health of loved ones. When you are snoring so loudly that those near you can get any sleep, it is a problem for everyone. Consider using un-medicated nasal strips to help control your snoring.

56.   To deal with snoring in a relationship, it's important to communicate honestly with your partner. If your snoring is keeping your significant other awake at night, the frustration can wear on both of you. Work together to find a solution to the problem, so you can stop snoring and strengthen your relationship at the same time.

57.   In order to reduce snoring, do not drink alcohol during the 4 to 5 hours before you go to sleep. Alcohol has a sedative effect and will make your throat muscles relax too much when you sleep. This can contribute to snoring, even if you do not normally have a tendency to snore.

58.   Moderate the amount of dairy intake during your meals if you want to reduce snoring when you

rest. Dairy can expedite the formation of mucus in your body, which can clog your airways and make it tough to breathe at night. Curtail your dairy consumption at all costs to breathe freely as the night wears on.

59.   Avoid taking anything before bed if you have a snoring problem. Muscle relaxers, alcohol and other drugs can loosen your throat muscles. If this happens, they could collapse inward, causing an obstruction in your air passage, which may result in snoring. If you have to drink something before bedtime, make it water.

60.   If all of your remedies fail, one of the things that you can do is seek professional advice from a doctor. There are many different types of surgeries that you can undergo to increase your air passages so that you can breathe more efficiently at night. Get professional help if your snoring becomes a serious dilemma.

61.   Lose some weight if you want to stop snoring. Losing weight will significantly increase your ability to pass air through your air passageway. Being overweight can cause the space in this air passageway to narrow, and that will cause snoring that will disturb both you and your family.

62.   Losing weight is a good step to take in order to stop snoring at night while you are asleep. Extra weight restricts breathing, especially extra weight around the neck. Maintain a balanced diet, exercise, and lose a few pounds to help remedy your breathing and snoring issues.

63.   Sleeping while having your head raised higher than the rest of your body will help prevent snoring. You can prop the whole front of the bed up, or you can elevate your head and part of your upper body. Do not just elevate your head, as this actually restricts breathing further.

64.   Learn about Dreamweaver, Photoshop, and other design software that can help you with web design projects. If you are unaware of these programs or what they do, invest some time in learning them and their uses.

65.   Chronic allergies are a common cause of snoring in many people. When the nasal passages are swollen and full of mucous, it forces you to breathe through your mouth, causing you to snore. Check with your doctor for medications that can treat your allergies, and thus, may end your snoring.

66.   To help you prevent snoring you should change the position in which you sleep. When you sleep on

your back it is said to cause people to snore. So switching positions can reduce or eliminate snoring. Instead of sleeping on your back, try sleeping on your side or stomach to prevent you from snoring.

67.   If you want to lower your chances of snoring when you sleep, you need to change bad lifestyle habits. Bad lifestyle habits such as smoking, or excessive caffeine can lead to people snoring. Those poor lifestyle choices put strain on your breathing which can make you snore while you sleep.

68.   A good tip for people who wish to eliminate their snoring problem is to stop using any sort of tranquilizer. While it may help you sleep, the muscles in your mouth and throat will be extremely relaxed which actually promotes snoring. Keep them out of your system if you wish to stop snoring.

69.   If you have a snoring problem, avoid sleeping on your back. This position makes snoring more likely because of the way the soft palate and base of the tongue rest at the back of your mouth. Instead, sleep on your side. You are less likely to snore in this position and your quality of sleep will likely improve.

70.   Take care of your allergies to alleviate snoring. Many times, snoring is caused by an allergy to dust mites, pet fur, or other allergen. The allergy can cause your nasal and throat passages to swell, leading to a rattling snore. Taking an over the counter medication can help, or see your doctor to find the best treatment.

71.   Try not to take any medications that contain sedatives, if you want to stop snoring. Sedatives are known to relax the throat muscles and when these muscles are too relaxed, snoring occurs. If you medications have sedatives, speak with your doctor about switching to a similar medication that does not have a sedative.

72.   A way to avoid the snoring that comes with extremely deep sleep is to develop and keep a steady sleep routine. If your body is accustomed to resting at a certain time, that sleep will be calmer, and you'll snore less. Getting a regular 8 hours a night, at the same time each night, will make sleeping more beneficial (and quieter for those around you).

73.   Try to to avoid consuming alcohol right before bed. Alcohol does help you relax; the problem is drinking alcohol right before bed causes the muscles of your airway to relax too much. This over

relaxation causes snoring which you may not notice. but, people around you will definitely be disturbed.

74.   Try using a pillow to elevate your head when you are a chronic snorer. Purchase a thicker pillow or just simply use more than one pillow. You may already have around the house. This will ensure you open up your airways and ensure that your partner also gets a good nights sleep.

75.   To help alleviate snoring, try to use over-the-counter snoring aids that help to open your airway. Snoring is often caused by the airway being constricted. By simply changing how you breathe, snoring can be relieved. There are many products available that can help open your airway, without needing to take any pills.

76.   In order to reduce snoring at night, work to clear your nasal passages before going to bed. You can take a nasal decongestant (pill or spray), or sleep with a neti pot next to your bed for a more organic solution. Getting the mucus out of your passages will make it less likely that you will snore.

77.   There are several methods to help you stop snoring by building throat muscles. One of these requires you to stand in front of the mirror and open your mouth. Work the muscle in the rear of

your throat. If you're contracting that muscle correctly, you'll see the uvula bobbing up and down -- and you'll stop snoring.

78.   It should not be surprising to read that losing weight will help to reduce snoring. This is common advice for snorers and the reasons are simple. If you have extra fatty tissue around your neck, this restricts your airway. Your muscles are weaker and your throat is more likely to relax and then, close up when you fall asleep.

79.   Make sure that you try to moderate the amount of exercise within an hour of going to bed. Exercising this close to bedtime can leave you breathless as you try to sleep. The lack of breathing will constrict the airways to the mouth and nose, thus resulting in snoring throughout the night.

80.   Try not to go to bed until at least a couple of hours after you have consumed a particularly large meal. One effect of a full stomach is that it pushes up against your diaphragm making it less flexible and restricting its normal range of movement. This can translate into increased snoring.

81.   A tennis ball could be the cure for your snoring! You can sew a pocket inside the back of your night shirt for the ball, or simply pin the ball onto the

back of the shirt. While you are sleeping, you will naturally turn on your side when you feel the tennis ball on your back. As sleeping bilaterally ameliorates snoring issues, this tip may be invaluable to you!

32.   You will probably not be as likely to snore if you avoid sleeping on your back. If it is troubling you that you cannot figure out a way to not fall asleep on your back, consider fastening a big object on the back of what you are wearing to sleep. Using this technique will cause you to experience mild discomfort if you rollover onto your back while sleeping.

33.   You should not eat or drink dairy products right before you go to sleep. They can cause excess mucus build-up, which in turn causes different breathing, resulting in snoring. There are plenty of other times throughout the day to eat dairy products, so cut out that ice cream before you go to bed.

34.   If you notice that you are snoring more and have put on a few pounds, you can solve the problem by losing the extra weight. Being overweight can cause your soft palate to encroach on your breathing passageway, which causes snoring.

85.   Smoking can be a factor in your snoring levels. Quitting can ease this. When you smoke, your throat's back tissues may become irritated and cause your throat to swell. Swelling in the throat is one of the major causes of snoring.

86.   If you want to stop snoring, try sleeping on your side. When you sleep on your stomach it can put pressure on your neck region. This can cause snoring. in addition, sleeping on your back restricts air flow to your body, also causing snoring. This is why sleeping on your left or right side is considered to be the best position if snoring is a problem.

87.   If you are finding that snoring is being an issue to you, have a look at the scales and see if you are currently overweight. If you are carrying excess weight, then you need to look at getting rid of it so that you can relieve the pressure which is being put on your airways.

88.   Snoring is common for people who sleep on their backs; however, it's hard to sleep on your side if your habit is to roll on your back. Stitch a tennis ball into the rear of your pajama shirt -- when you roll onto your back, the nuisance will push you back to your side, and you'll stop snoring.

89.   Drinking alcohol too close to bedtime can result in snoring. This happens because alcohol tends to relax the throat muscles, which leads to tightened airways. As a result, snoring is more likely to occur. The best way to avoid snoring due to alcohol consumption is to stop drinking spirits at least 5 to 6 hours before bedtime.

90.   Do not eat a meal just before bed. Having a full stomach can put pressure on your lungs and throat, which can in turn cause snoring. To stop this from happening, do not eat for roughly an hour before you go to bed. Not only will you sleep quietly, but your sleep will likely be more restful.

91.   To stop snoring, you should first look at your pillows. Many people fail to realize that proper support from pillows can impact whether you snore or not. Elevating the head can help keep your airway open to reduce and prevent snoring. This is a very simple and easy way to help snoring.

92.   While you are sleeping, it helps to have your head elevated. A thick, firm pillow offers extra support for your head and neck. Alternatively, you can simply use extra pillows. With your head in this elevated position, you'll be able to breathe better, which can diminish or eliminate your snoring.

93.   Blow your nose well before you go to bed. Often snoring is caused by a buildup of mucous in your nose. A stopped-up nose typically causes you to open your mouth during your sleep in order to breathe. When you breathe through your mouth you snore so keep some tissue at the side of your bed to prevent the problem before it starts.

94.   If you eat or drink any dairy products before you go to bed at night it will make your snoring worse. Dairy can produce extra mucus, and this will cause your airways to be clogged up. This leads to snore and a horrible night's sleep for you and the person you sleep with every night.

95.   You can cut back on the amount of snoring you do by giving up smoking. If you find it difficult to give up smoking, you can enjoy some benefits by avoiding tobacco for the few hours before bed. Smoking reduces the amount of space available in your airway by making your throat swell. An inflamed throat and narrow pathways will cause snoring; therefore, not smoking can lead to less swelling of the throat and less snoring

96.   If your snoring seems severe, you should speak to your doctor. You will probably need a sleep study to determine if you have sleep apnea. If you do, the doctor will probably recommend that you

use a CPAP machine at nighttime. The CPAP machine forces air into your airways to keep them open. This keeps you from snoring and it also makes sure you are well oxygenated.

97.   Stop smoking or, at least, abstain from smoking right before bedtime. Smoking has many health impacts. One of the more annoying is its contribution to snoring. Your airway is irritated by the smoke and can become swollen. This can cause you to snore more than you would without the irritation.

98.   An adjustment in your sleeping position may be just what you need to stop snoring. Snoring is more likely to occur when you sleep on your back. Sleeping on your side can put an end to your snoring problem. Try to avoid sleeping on your stomach, it strains your neck.

99.   If you have allergies and snore, investigate your allergies as a source of the snoring. Allergies that go untreated can make the nasal passage swell; when that happens, you will have no choice but to inhale and exhale through your mouth. Snoring is a common result of this behavior. Try allergy medications that you get over the counter and see if they work for you. If not, you're doctor may need to prescribe you something.

100.   If you or a loved one has noticed that you have a snoring problem, you should make an appointment to be evaluated in a sleep study. You may have sleep apnea, a condition where the esophagus closes and causes breathing problems such as snoring. If you have sleep apnea, you may be eligible for a c-pap machine that will create positive air flow while you sleep, curing snoring as well as breathing related problems.

101.   If you smoke, it may be wise to quit smoking to help you stop snoring. Smoking can irritate your throat, and cause it to swell. Swelling of the throat is often the cause of snoring.

102.   If snoring has become a nighttime concern, then it is time to give dairy products such as milk, yogurt or cheese a miss before you go to sleep each night. This is because the dairy products can cause mucus to build up near your breathing passages, and this will trigger off snoring.

103.   Stick to a regular bedtime, and practice good sleep habits in general to reduce the incidence of snoring. If you go to bed overtired, sleep erratic hours, or have other bad sleep habits, you may sleep very deeply which relaxes the muscles in the back of

your throat more than usual. This can contribute to snoring.

104.   If you snore, sew a tennis ball on the backside of your shirt. The reason for this is that it will prevent you from sleeping on your back, which is the main position that a person snores in. If you do not have a tennis ball, you could use a baseball.

105.   If you are dealing with allergies, you are probably going to be suffering from congestion, making it more likely you will snore as you sleep. Your nasal passages and your airway will become congested if you have allergies. This congestion can easily lead to heavy snoring. One suggestion on how to fight this is to use a decongestant before bed in order to have a more peaceful night's sleep.

106.   Buy a new pillow to help with your snoring. Sometimes all you need to stop snoring is to change pillows. Some pillows restrict your breathing passages. This makes you open your mouth in compensation and, when you breathe through your mouth, you start snoring. Try using a firmer pillow and one that elevates your head somewhat more than your old pillow.

107.   In order to reduce snoring, do not drink alcohol during the 4 to 5 hours before you go to sleep.

Alcohol has a sedative effect and will make your throat muscles relax too much when you sleep. This can contribute to snoring, even if you do not normally have a tendency to snore.

108.   Stop smoking to stop snoring. When you inhale tobacco smoke into your lungs, irritants are produced that affect your airway and nasal membranes. The resulting inflammation causes your throat to narrow and contributes to your snoring. Try not to smoke before going to bed, or better yet give it up all together.

109.   Use a good pillow which provides adequate elevation for your head during sleep. To combat snoring, which is caused by constricted air passageways, it is essential that you keep those airways open and unobstructed. Make sure the pillow you use is doing a good job of keeping your head sufficiently elevated so that you can get better rest at night.

110.   Try not to go to bed until at least a couple of hours after you have consumed a particularly large meal. One effect of a full stomach is that it pushes up against your diaphragm making it less flexible and restricting its normal range of movement. This can translate into increased snoring.

111.   As with so many other health issues, obesity definitely increases the occurrences of snoring. A recent increase in snoring could easily be the result of a recent increase in weight. Even if losing that weight does not completely solve your snoring problem, you can only gain from getting more fit.

112.   Interestingly, it is possible to eliminate snoring using a tennis ball. All you have to do is use a safety pin to attach the tennis ball to the rear of your pajamas prior to bedtime. When you sleep, you probably will turn over and feel the ball up against your back. Snoring can reduce your snoring a lot.

113.   You should avoid alcohol, sedative or sleeping pills before going to bed. These things can make your throat muscles and tissues to relax and obstruct your breathing which will cause snoring. You may feel that your snoring is causing you to lose sleep so you take a sleeping pill. But this will only make the snoring worse so you should avoid them.

114.   You can minimize or eliminate your nightly snoring with the help of nasal or throat sprays. Some sprays are designed to relieve congestion in your nose and throat which allows you to breathe easier. Other sprays are more like a lubricant that

moisturizes your dry, irritated nasal passages and throat which will reduce or eliminate snoring.

115.   In efforts to help yourself stop snoring, stop smoking cigarettes. Maybe you never have smoked a cigarette, but if you have, they affect your respiratory system in an unmatched way. Stop smoking cigarettes to help you stop snoring at night, and also for your general health. Smoking is not good for you in any way.

116.   Visiting the dentist could be in order if you want to reduce your snoring. The dentist can give you a mouth-guard that is constructed by using a mold. This is a mouth-guard you wear at night. It is designed to pull the lower jaw forward, keeping your throat's tissues from collapsing while you sleep, which is what makes you snore.

117.   Consider learning how to play a juice harp as part of your fight against snoring. This instrument is also called a mouth harp. It is placed inside your mouth and, as you pluck the sound tone of the instrument, you variously tighten and loosen your mouth muscles to produce different sounds as the vibrations from the tine resonate inside the chamber of your mouth.

118.   If you want to stop snoring, try sleeping on your side. When you sleep on your stomach it can put pressure on your neck region. This can cause snoring. in addition, sleeping on your back restricts air flow to your body, also causing snoring. This is why sleeping on your left or right side is considered to be the best position if snoring is a problem.

119.   Not eating a large meal close to bedtime is one of the best ways to prevent snoring. When your stomach is too full, it can makes it's way up to your diaphragm, thus, limiting your breathing and causing snoring. Stick with big meals at dinnertime and have a light snack instead before bed.

120.   To help ease your snoring, try falling asleep with your head in a slightly raised position. A thicker pillow will provide more support for your head. Also, you can stack two thinner pillows atop one another. Using this technique will help to open your throat, allowing more air flow, resulting in less snoring.

121.   If you snore, you may want to consider using nasal strips. These strips resemble a Band-Aid. However, they are different than a normal Band-Aid. Nasal strips are made to keep nasal passages open and functioning normally. This will make it

easier for you to breath from the nose, and when that happens, your snoring will decrease.

122.   To deal with snoring in a relationship, it's important to communicate honestly with your partner. If your snoring is keeping your significant other awake at night, the frustration can wear on both of you. Work together to find a solution to the problem, so you can stop snoring and strengthen your relationship at the same time.

123.   There are several methods to help you stop snoring by building throat muscles. One of these requires you to stand in front of the mirror and open your mouth. Work the muscle in the rear of your throat. If you're contracting that muscle correctly, you'll see the uvula bobbing up and down -- and you'll stop snoring.

124.   Drinking water is a great way to create a smooth passageway for the air in your body. During the course of the day, drink at least eight glasses of water to maximize hydration. Water will help you to feel refreshed and can aid in breathing freely at night, reducing the chance that you will snore.

125.   Try to lose a few pounds if you want to see a decrease in snoring. Extra weight around your airway can cause an increase in pressure, which can

lead to snoring. This pressure can cause your airways to constrict or partially collapse as you sleep. Your snoring may be improved if you lose even a couple of pounds.

126.   Refrain from sleeping on a mattress that you sink into or is slanted. This will cause your body to be at an angle, which can put tension on your air passages during the night. Try to find a mattress that is parallel to the ground so that you can breathe efficiently without snoring.

127.   Keep a glass of water and a box of Kleenex next to your bed. If you are waking up at night due to snoring, drink a bit of water and blow your nose. Many times this will lubricate both your nose and throat passageways and can eliminate your snoring, at least for a few hours.

128.   Allergies are a common cause of snoring that can be effectively treated. If allergies go untreated, they cause a swelling of your nasal passages and this keeps you from breathing through your nose. Snoring is almost certainly going to be the result. An over-the-counter antihistamine may help, or visit your doctor if your allergies are severe enough to warrant a prescription.

129.   You should not eat or drink dairy products right before you go to sleep. They can cause excess mucus build-up, which in turn causes different breathing, resulting in snoring. There are plenty of other times throughout the day to eat dairy products, so cut out that ice cream before you go to bed.

130.   Eating a large meal right before you go to bed is never a good idea. The fuller your stomach, the more it will be pushing on your diaphragm, restricting your breathing. If you must eat right before bed, eat a small snack, and of course avoid any dairy products as well.

131.   Consider learning how to play a juice harp as part of your fight against snoring. This instrument is also called a mouth harp. It is placed inside your mouth and, as you pluck the sound tone of the instrument, you variously tighten and loosen your mouth muscles to produce different sounds as the vibrations from the tine resonate inside the chamber of your mouth.

132.   Snoring can take a toll on your health because it interrupts your normal sleep patterns so that you never get all the rest you need. While you are looking for a cure to your snoring problem, be sure to get enough rest, even napping once in a while.

This will help to keep your energy level up, and fatigue to a minimum.

133.   If you want to lower your chances of snoring when you sleep, you need to change bad lifestyle habits. Bad lifestyle habits such as smoking, or excessive caffeine can lead to people snoring. Those poor lifestyle choices put strain on your breathing which can make you snore while you sleep.

134.   Changing sleeping positions can help stop snoring. Many people sleep on their backs since gravity forces their heads down, which closes the throat. You may find it easier to sleep on your side, because it reduces the pressure on your neck, as well as your likelihood of snoring.

135.   "Fish face" may sound silly, but it could help you to stop snoring. Repeatedly making these faces can make your throat and facial muscles stronger. To perform the exercise purse your lips and draw your cheeks in. Try moving your lips like a fish. For best results, do this a few times each day.

136.   To stop snoring, go on a weight loss regimen if you are currently overweight. Fat is intruding on the available space for your air passages, and those narrower passages are causing you to snore. If you

get rid of the fat, your passages will be able to open fully, and you can stop snoring.

137.   If you're affected by congestion caused by allergies or anything else, snoring becomes a greater probability when you're sleeping. When you are congested, your nasal passages will become constricted, blocking airflow and causing you to snore. One option is to take a decongestant before your bedtime; however, you should only use products that are formulated for nighttime use. Otherwise, it may be difficult to fall asleep.

138.   Buy a new pillow to help with your snoring. Sometimes all you need to stop snoring is to change pillows. Some pillows restrict your breathing passages. This makes you open your mouth in compensation and, when you breathe through your mouth, you start snoring. Try using a firmer pillow and one that elevates your head somewhat more than your old pillow.

139.   In order to reduce snoring at night, work to clear your nasal passages before going to bed. You can take a nasal decongestant (pill or spray), or sleep with a neti pot next to your bed for a more organic solution. Getting the mucus out of your passages will make it less likely that you will snore.

140.   In order to reduce snoring, do not drink alcohol during the 4 to 5 hours before you go to sleep. Alcohol has a sedative effect and will make your throat muscles relax too much when you sleep. This can contribute to snoring, even if you do not normally have a tendency to snore.

141.   Lose as much excess weight as possible. Extra weight does not just show up in your thighs, it can make your throat narrower. This can cause snoring and sleep apnea. Even a 10 pound loss can help open up the passageway in your throat. The more wide open it is, the better you will sleep.

142.   If you are bothered by nightly snoring, consider any drugs that you may be taking as a possible cause. Some medications dry out your nasal membranes, which can restrict airflow and cause snoring. There are also medications designed to sedate; they end up relaxing your throat so that airflow is restricted during sleep.

143.   Stop smoking to stop snoring. When you inhale tobacco smoke into your lungs, irritants are produced that affect your airway and nasal membranes. The resulting inflammation causes your throat to narrow and contributes to your snoring. Try not to smoke before going to bed, or better yet give it up all together.

144.   You could often lessen your snoring using a tennis ball. Fasten the ball onto the back of clothing before you are about to go to sleep. The discomfort you feel from the tennis ball will naturally cause you to turn to sleep on your side. Side sleepers tend not to snore as the airway is unobstructed in that position.

145.   If you are overweight, implement a diet regimen to cut down the excess fat on your body. This fat, especially in your neck region, plays a large role in constricting the air from traveling throughout your body. Losing weight will not only improve your health but can reduce your snoring as well.

146.   Use nasal strips to help you sleep. Nasal strips expand the nostrils to facilitate air flow, which reduces snoring. This will allow not only you to sleep well, but you also won't be disturbing your family as you slumber. Purchase brand-name nasal strips at your local grocery store and apply them before you go to bed.

147.   If you haven't been able to treat your snoring, try scheduling an appointment with your dentist. He can make a mold of the inside of your mouth, then use it to make a mouth-guard. This mouth guard will help push the lower jaw forward, which will

keep the muscles from narrowing during sleep. This constriction of tissues will cause snoring.

148.   One simple piece of advice to snorers is to make sure you are drinking plenty of water each day. While this may not be a cure for snoring, it will keep air passages and soft palate moist and reduce any mucous that may build up during the day. Excess mucous can cause snoring.

149.   Attempt to cleanse your nasal cavities before bed. Many people that snore simply have issues with their nose or sinuses, so using a decongestant right before bed is a simple solution. An easy way to do this is to inhale hot steam for a minute or two. This will clear things up naturally if you are leery of using medication.

150.   Snoring can not only be annoying for you but can also be annoying to anybody that has to sleep near you. Nasal strips are an effective way to reduce snoring; you simply place them on your nose at bedtime. You and your family will sleep better at night if you wear one of these, even though they are the most attractive thing to wear.

151.   If you want to stop snoring, don't consume alcohol just before bed. While alcohol is OK to have with dinner or even later in the evening, if you

have it just before bed, it will make all of your muscles relax -- including those that keep your nasal passages fully open. You'll have less air flow, and you'll snore.

152.   Quit smoking, or drastically cut back to stop snoring. Smoking causes all sorts of damage to your respiratory system and other parts of your body. If you are a heavy smoker, smoking might actually be the cause of your snoring problem. Quit smoking to stop the snoring and live a healthier lifestyle.

153.   Sleep more upright. Elevating your upper body can relieve both gravity and pressure, allowing you to get a full night's rest without snoring. Use pillows or put some bricks under the headboard. Even just a slight elevation can stop you from snoring, so try it out and see what height works best for you.

154.   A way to avoid the snoring that comes with extremely deep sleep is to develop and keep a steady sleep routine. If your body is accustomed to resting at a certain time, that sleep will be calmer, and you'll snore less. Getting a regular 8 hours a night, at the same time each night, will make sleeping more beneficial (and quieter for those around you).

155.   Unstop your nose to quit snoring. Snoring can be an embarrassing problem. It can relate to a number of factors, not the least of which is nasal congestion. One way to address snoring is to talk to your doctor about decongestants. These medications can be a very effective remedy not just for the embarrassment of snoring but also for the underlying condition.

156.   Consult your physician if you snore on a regular basis, because you may be suffering from a sleep disorder called sleep apnea. People with this disorder actually stop breathing for a period of time while sleeping and may wake up briefly in order to resume breathing. This can result in daytime fatigue. Sleep apnea can be treated, so it is important to receive medical intervention.

157.   If you want to stop snoring, talk to your dentist or physician about a mouth guard. The purpose of the guard is to keep your teeth together, and to ensure that the lower jaw muscles do not relax so much that your air passageways slacken, and snoring starts again. That's the last thing you want!

158.   In order to reduce snoring, do not drink alcohol during the 4 to 5 hours before you go to sleep. Alcohol has a sedative effect and will make your throat muscles relax too much when you sleep. This

can contribute to snoring, even if you do not normally have a tendency to snore.

159.   Talk to your doctor about prescribing something to help you quit snoring. While medication performance varies among different users, some snorers have found their snoring is greatly reduced when they use medications that are hailed as anti-snoring remedies. These remedies come in various forms ranging from pills to nasal sprays.

160.   Believe it or not, the normal aging process can contribute to the onset of snoring. As we become older, the muscle tone in the airway becomes narrower and the throat can lose significant muscle tone. Talk to your doctor if snoring is becoming a problem so that you can avoid health issues related to this annoying condition.

161.   Some basic exercises can cut down on snoring. Try doing some throat exercises for about 15 or 30 minutes to keep your throat muscles from collapsing. You will execute this by voicing vowel sounds and repeated curling of your tongue. This strengthens your upper respiratory area, as well as the muscles.

162.   There are some hereditary abnormalities that a person can be born with that increases the

likelihood of him or her snoring at night. Also, men have a narrow nasal passageway compared to women, increasing their chances of snoring more than women. Learn what you can do in order to prevent snoring according to your unique situation.

163.   Eat a light dinner if you are trying to stop your snoring. When you have a heavy meal, your stomach expands and fills more of your abdominal cavity. If you have less food in your stomach before you lay down, this will increase the capacity your lungs have for taking in oxygen.

164.   In order to eliminate your snoring, you may need to ask your doctor or dentist about getting a mouth guard. These things can hold your teeth together and prevent your lower jaw muscles from being too loose when you are sleeping. This method is one of the most effective ones for eliminating snoring.

165.   Snoring can take a toll on your health because it interrupts your normal sleep patterns so that you never get all the rest you need. While you are looking for a cure to your snoring problem, be sure to get enough rest, even napping once in a while. This will help to keep your energy level up, and fatigue to a minimum.

166.   Refrain from consuming dairy products late at night if you want to reduce snoring. If you eat dairy, mucus might build up in your throat and cause snoring. The dairy that produces mucus may cause your airways to be blocked, which could lead to excessive snoring.

167.   If you regularly take prescription muscle relaxers or pain medications, you might be faced with chronic snoring. If at all possible, avoid taking these medications in the hours before you get ready for bed. These drugs cause your muscles to become more relaxed, especially in your airways. As a result, it becomes more difficult to breathe, which leads to snoring.

168.   To reduce snoring, avoid drinking milk or eating dairy products before going to sleep. Warm milk was once thought to be a helpful remedy to drink before sleeping; however, if you snore, dairy increases mucous production. Over production of mucous often makes snoring much worse. By avoiding dairy before you go to sleep, you help keep your airway clear.

169.   Nasal strips may help alleviate snoring. Nasal strips strongly resemble Band-Aids. On the other hand, they work in a very different manner. Their purpose is to make sure your nasal passages are

open. This facilitates breathing through your nose, and when you do that, you won't snore.

170.   To help reduce snoring, losing weight can be beneficial. People fail to realize that weight gain has an impact on breathing. By losing weight, you actually increase your air passage. Excessive weight impacts the comfort of your sleep. Losing weight is a basic way to help rid you of snoring and has many other health benefits.

171.   If you want to stop snoring, upgrade to a pillow that is a bit firmer. Soft pillows relax your throat muscles, which narrows your airway. Because air is having a harder time getting through, you'll start snoring. It may be helpful to rest your head on a firmer pillow.

172.   To keep yourself from snoring at night, turn on a humidifier before you go to sleep. The warm moisture will keep mucus from gathering in your throat, and will keep your whole nasal system moist. These two factors will keep your nasal passageways clearer, and keep you from snoring all night.

173.   Treat your allergies if you have a tendency to snore at night. If you are congested or your respiratory system is irritated, you will be more likely to snore when you go to sleep. Use a

decongestant or an antihistamine to treat your allergies, and keep your airway clear at night.

174.   Use a good pillow which provides adequate elevation for your head during sleep. To combat snoring, which is caused by constricted air passageways, it is essential that you keep those airways open and unobstructed. Make sure the pillow you use is doing a good job of keeping your head sufficiently elevated so that you can get better rest at night.

175.   Nose strips can be an inexpensive solution to try. They are a thin strip of material with an adhesive on the back. Once attached to the bridge of your nose, they hold the nasal passages open and allow you to breath more easily during the night and can eliminate snoring for many.

176.   Try to establish a regular schedule for sleep. Experienced snorers and their mates have observed that when you sleep at unpredictable times you have an increased propensity for snoring. Set a definitive time to go to bed and adhere to that schedule every night. Avoid activities like playing electronic games that might keep you from getting to sleep at the defined time.

177.   Do some tongue exercises. A common cause of snoring is the tongue falling back toward your throat and blocking the air passage. Doing tongue exercises can strengthen the tongue to tone this muscle. Stick your tongue straight out as far as you can, then move it from left to right, up and down.

178.   To minimize snoring, try to eat a large breakfast and lunch during the day. This will force you to have a smaller dinner, which is very beneficial towards maintaining a high comfort level when you sleep at night. The more comfortable you are when you rest, the less of a chance for you to snore.

179.   Refrain from eating rich foods such as pizza and cake in the hours leading up to bed. These foods can clog your airways and make it harder for you to breathe at night. The better you are able to take in air, the more flowing your breathing will be at night, minimizing snoring.

180.   Wearing nasal strips while you are sleeping ensures a continuous opening of your nasal air passages, which can help alleviate much of your snoring. Try wearing nasal strips at night while you are sleeping, and see how they work for you. Using them in conjunction with other tips has been known to significantly reduce how much a person snores.

181.   One of the oldest methods to prevent snoring is the use of a chin strap. Their design has changed over the years so that the new ones are quite comfortable. They keep your mouth from opening at night so that are not breathing through your mouth. Thus, you must breathe through your nose, which keeps you from snoring.

182.   If you snore, try going to the dentist to see if they can help. It is easy for him to make a molded mouth guard for you. When you wear this mouth-guard at night, it will position your jaw forward just up to the point where your throat muscles will not collapse while you sleep, thus eliminating a possible cause of your snoring.

183.   If you are pregnant and notice that you are developing a snoring problem, be sure to mention it to your doctor. The excess weight and hormonal changes of pregnancy can cause changes in the throat that can contribute to this irritating noise. It is important to check with your physician to be sure snoring doesn't deprive your baby of oxygen.

184.   Most people snore during their deepest sleep while lying on their back. Usually, it is not a problem unless the snoring disturbs their sleeping partner, in which case, they will probably be

awakened and be asked to roll on their side. This action is probably the first and oldest cure for snoring.

185.   If you have a snoring problem, avoid sleeping on your back. This position makes snoring more likely because of the way the soft palate and base of the tongue rest at the back of your mouth. Instead, sleep on your side. You are less likely to snore in this position and your quality of sleep will likely improve.

186.   If you regularly use cigarettes and other tobacco products, you probably also snore. The ingredients in these products dries out the mucosal membranes in your nose, mouth and airway, which leads to difficulty breathing and loud snoring. If at all possible, do not smoke cigarettes within five hours of your bedtime as the smoke will cause your airway to become inflamed.

187.   If you snore while you are pregnant, make a trip to the doctor immediately. While it is very common for pregnant women to snore during their pregnancies, you should learn about how this problem can affect your baby and its oxygen levels. To ensure that your baby is not deprived of oxygen, consult your doctor.

188.   A way to avoid the snoring that comes with extremely deep sleep is to develop and keep a steady sleep routine. If your body is accustomed to resting at a certain time, that sleep will be calmer, and you'll snore less. Getting a regular 8 hours a night, at the same time each night, will make sleeping more beneficial (and quieter for those around you).

189.   Excessive snoring can sometimes keep you from getting a restful night's sleep, but if you do snore never take sleeping pills. Sleeping pills cause every muscle in your body to relax, including the muscles in your jaw and neck. This will only serve to make your snoring problems worse and severe problems like sleep apnea can develop.

190.   Don't drink alcoholic beverages before going to bed. The very reason you might be tempted to have a nighttime drink, the fact that you want to relax, can cause you to snore. When your muscles relax because of the alcohol, so do your air passages. As your air passages become restricted, you snore.

191.   Treat your allergies if you have a tendency to snore at night. If you are congested or your respiratory system is irritated, you will be more likely to snore when you go to sleep. Use a

decongestant or an antihistamine to treat your allergies, and keep your airway clear at night.

192.   Make your bedroom as allergy-proof as you can. If you suffer from allergies, it is important that you try to prevent congestion due to allergic reactions from affecting your sleep. Congestion during sleep leads to snoring. Remove as many of your allergy triggers as possible from your bedroom in order to give yourself the best chance of enjoying a peaceful night's rest.

193.   Dairy foods may be causing your snoring, whether or not you have lactose intolerance. Dairy products stimulate your body to produce more phlegm, which can then fill your nose and throat and make it difficult to breathe. If you usually have warm milk at bedtime, try hot mint or cinnamon tea, instead! That will help you relax and open your airways!

194.   One tennis ball could often help reduce your snoring. To use this method pin a tennis ball onto the back of the pajamas you will be wearing that night. When you sleep, you probably will turn over and feel the ball up against your back. Side-sleeping will cut snoring sounds significantly.

195.   If all of your remedies fail, one of the things that you can do is seek professional advice from a doctor. There are many different types of surgeries that you can undergo to increase your air passages so that you can breathe more efficiently at night. Get professional help if your snoring becomes a serious dilemma.

196.   You can cut down on snoring by being more aware of what you consume before bed. You should avoid dairy products such as milk, ice cream or yogurt. These foods cause the production of thick mucus which can obstruct the throat and nasal passages. This will cause snoring. So, it is best for you to avoid these food before going to bed.

197.   Take a good hot shower before going to bed. Not only will it relax you and help you get to sleep, the steam from the shower will moisturize and open your respiratory passages. When you are dry inside you are more likely to snore. The steam will remedy that problem.

198.   Use nasal strips to help you sleep. Nasal strips expand the nostrils to facilitate air flow, which reduces snoring. This will allow not only you to sleep well, but you also won't be disturbing your family as you slumber. Purchase brand-name nasal

strips at your local grocery store and apply them before you go to bed.

199.   If you notice that you are snoring more and have put on a few pounds, you can solve the problem by losing the extra weight. Being overweight can cause your soft palate to encroach on your breathing passageway, which causes snoring.

200.   Avoid drinking alcohol within 5 hours of bedtime. Alcohol, along with other sedative drugs, causes the muscles at the back of the throat to relax. When these muscles relax, you are more apt to snore. Stay away from those nightcaps--you may actually sleep more soundly if you do not drink before bed.

201.   You may want to think about getting a mouth device to prevent breathing through your mouth when you sleep. Breathing through your mouth, and not your nose, can cause snoring. These mouth devices block breathing through your mouth and encourage you to breathe through your nose instead. Speak with your doctor about this option.

202.   To stop snoring, try getting a firmer pillow. Soft pillows can relax the throat muscles, which narrow the air passages. This constriction makes it more

difficult to push air through the airways, which leads to snoring. A pillow that is firmer can help with keeping your airway open.

203.   To deal with snoring in a relationship, it's important to communicate honestly with your partner. If your snoring is keeping your significant other awake at night, the frustration can wear on both of you. Work together to find a solution to the problem, so you can stop snoring and strengthen your relationship at the same time.

204.   Try to lose a few pounds if you want to see a decrease in snoring. If you have extra fat, especially around your neck, this will put an increased amount of pressure directly on your airways. This can cause your muscles to become lax late in the night, leading to an increased snoring problem. You can see decreased snoring by just losing a few pounds.

205.   Sleep in an elevated position to help reduce your snoring. Sleeping in a horizontal position can put more pressure on your airway causing it to close. By elevating your whole upper body and not just your head, you can relieve this extra pressure. Try propping your whole torso up on pillows or putting some blocks beneath your bedposts at the head of your bed.

206.   Keep a glass of water and a box of Kleenex next to your bed. If you are waking up at night due to snoring, drink a bit of water and blow your nose. Many times this will lubricate both your nose and throat passageways and can eliminate your snoring, at least for a few hours.

207.   An adjustment in your sleeping position may be just what you need to stop snoring. Snoring is more likely to occur when you sleep on your back. Sleeping on your side can put an end to your snoring problem. Try to avoid sleeping on your stomach, it strains your neck.

208.   If you want to stop snoring when you sleep, you should sleep on your side. Sleeping on your back instigates snoring, and sleeping on your stomach just hurts your neck. Sleeping on your side helps you rest peacefully, without having to worry about snoring as much. Give it a try!

209.   Alcohol and sleeping pills need to be avoided if you are trying to keep from snoring at night. They relax your muscles, and if your throat muscles are too relaxed, snoring is much more likely. Do not drink alcohol or take sleeping pills before bedtime, as this can also cause sleep apnea as well, which is a very dangerous condition.

210.   Try using certain essential oils to help you with you snoring problem. Peppermint oil or eucalyptus oil are just two of the essential oils that can reduce nasal congestion. This can make it easy to breathe and you may not snore. Try them out the next time your sinuses feel blocked.

211.   Eating a large meal right before you go to bed is never a good idea. The fuller your stomach, the more it will be pushing on your diaphragm, restricting your breathing. If you must eat right before bed, eat a small snack, and of course avoid any dairy products as well.

212.   One of the oldest methods to prevent snoring is the use of a chin strap. Their design has changed over the years so that the new ones are quite comfortable. They keep your mouth from opening at night so that are not breathing through your mouth. Thus, you must breathe through your nose, which keeps you from snoring.

213.   If you or your partner snores at night, do not sleep isolated from each other. Instead, help prevent snoring from happening as you select plan to deal with it. Sleeping away from each other just strains the relationship and restricts intimacy at night. Keep a healthy relationship, and eliminate snoring from your nightly routine.

214.   If you tend to snore, do not skip your breakfast
or lunch. If you fill yourself up with breakfast and
lunch, you will be less likely to overeat at
dinnertime. Lying down with an empty stomach will
help you breathe easier while sleeping.

215.   Consider learning how to play a juice harp as
part of your fight against snoring. This instrument is
also called a mouth harp. It is placed inside your
mouth and, as you pluck the sound tone of the
instrument, you variously tighten and loosen your
mouth muscles to produce different sounds as the
vibrations from the tine resonate inside the
chamber of your mouth.

216.   In order to decrease your snoring, you should
aim to steer away from consuming any type of dairy
products. This is because dairy can cause your
amount of mucus to build up prior to going to
sleep. This increased mucus can increase your
amount of snoring, so eliminating this mucus can
substantially help to eliminate snoring.

217.   One of the most common mistakes people
make during the evening is eating a huge meal in the
hours before their bedtime. If your stomach is filled
to capacity with food, it will take up more space and
press up against your diaphragm. This has the

unfortunate effect of making it difficult to breathe as you lie on your back.

218.   If you suffer from snoring, it is important that you not sleep on your back. This position narrows the airways in your throat, thus, reducing airflow. This lack of air can be a cause of snoring. It is recommended that you sleep on either your right or left side instead.

219.   Allergy and sinus sufferers tend to suffer from snoring. This is because you have too much congestion in your nose, so you are breathing in and out of your mouth when you are sleeping. If you have sinus or allergy issues, getting them properly treated could end your snoring as well.

220.   If snoring has become a nighttime concern, then it is time to give dairy products such as milk, yogurt or cheese a miss before you go to sleep each night. This is because the dairy products can cause mucus to build up near your breathing passages, and this will trigger off snoring.

221.   If your bedmate is a chronic snorer, it may become necessary to make certain adjustments to your schedules. Ask your snoring partner to wait until you have already fallen asleep before coming to bed. This way, you can fall asleep quickly and

may have a better chance of waking up being well-rested the next day.

222.   Quit smoking, or drastically cut back to stop snoring. Smoking causes all sorts of damage to your respiratory system and other parts of your body. If you are a heavy smoker, smoking might actually be the cause of your snoring problem. Quit smoking to stop the snoring and live a healthier lifestyle.

223.   To stop snoring, you should first look at your pillows. Many people fail to realize that proper support from pillows can impact whether you snore or not. Elevating the head can help keep your airway open to reduce and prevent snoring. This is a very simple and easy way to help snoring.

224.   Illegal drugs should never be used. Street drugs can dramatically increase your chances of snoring when you are asleep. Marijuana and other similar drugs are designed to create a feeling of relaxation. Pain killers bought on the street do the same thing. Even if these products relax you and help you go to sleep, they will not keep you from snoring.

225.   Prescription medications may be causing your snoring, speak with your doctor about it. There are prescription medicines that have snoring as a side effect. Medicines like pain killers, antihistamines,

sleeping pills and muscle relaxers all can restrict the airway. Restricted airways can cause you to snore.

226.   Do not consume dairy before going to bed. Dairy products may cause a build up of mucus in your respiratory system and this build up causes snoring. Do not eat ice cream, drink milk or consume any other dairy products before bed and this can help you avoid snoring.

227.   Blow your nose well before you go to bed. Often snoring is caused by a buildup of mucous in your nose. A stopped-up nose typically causes you to open your mouth during your sleep in order to breathe. When you breathe through your mouth you snore so keep some tissue at the side of your bed to prevent the problem before it starts.

228.   To help reduce snoring, losing weight can be beneficial. People fail to realize that weight gain has an impact on breathing. By losing weight, you actually increase your air passage. Excessive weight impacts the comfort of your sleep. Losing weight is a basic way to help rid you of snoring and has many other health benefits.

229.   To keep yourself from snoring at night, turn on a humidifier before you go to sleep. The warm moisture will keep mucus from gathering in your

throat, and will keep your whole nasal system moist. These two factors will keep your nasal passageways clearer, and keep you from snoring all night.

230.   Use nasal strips at night before you go to sleep. When you apply a strip to your nose, it will open both of your nostrils to let in more air. When the nasal passage is constricted, it can exacerbate the tendency to snore. Using nasal strips will result in a reduction in snoring.

231.   If nothing over the counter seems to be working for you, ask your doctor about a mouthpiece for the nighttime. IT will be fitted to your mouth and jaw. The idea is that it pulls your lower jaw slightly forward and allows your throat and airways to stay open wider as you sleep.

232.   To reduce snoring, learn to play the didgeridoo. The didgeridoo is a large Australian wind instrument. Studies have shown that playing the didgeridoo reduces snoring significantly. It strengthens the muscles in the upper throat and is also effective as a way to reduce sleep apnea, a potentially dangerous condition. Loud snorers often suffer from sleep apnea, abnormally low breathing during sleep.

233.   If you want to stop snoring when you sleep, you should sleep on your side. Sleeping on your back instigates snoring, and sleeping on your stomach just hurts your neck. Sleeping on your side helps you rest peacefully, without having to worry about snoring as much. Give it a try!

234.   Sleeping pills can contribute to snoring, so you might actually get a better night's sleep if you avoid them. The main effect of sleeping pills is to relax every one of your muscles. The one that keeps your nasal passage wide open also sags, enabling the passages to be narrow. Therefore, you are more likely to snore.

235.   If you suffer from chronic snoring, you may benefit from allergy testing. Allergies can clog the nasal passages and force you to breathe out of your mouth, which causes snoring. Finding out the causes of your allergies allows you to eliminate their sources. Also, you may benefit from taking a prescribed or over-the-counter antihistamine before bed.

236.   Avoid the consumption of alcohol before you go to bed in order to refrain from snoring. Because alcohol can relax the throat muscles, they may vibrate as air passes and cause snoring to occur. Allow several hours to pass after your last alcoholic

beverage before you go to sleep to minimize or eliminate snoring.

237.   To deal with snoring in a relationship, it's important to communicate honestly with your partner. If your snoring is keeping your significant other awake at night, the frustration can wear on both of you. Work together to find a solution to the problem, so you can stop snoring and strengthen your relationship at the same time.

238.   To cut back on your snoring, it's important to have a regular exercise regimen. When you're working your abs or your legs, your throat muscles are also working too. This makes your air passages firmer -- making them more likely to stay open and prevent snoring on your part.

239.   One of the best ways to eliminate snoring during the night is to cut down on your intake of alcohol during the day. Alcohol tends to tighten your airways, which will make it much harder to breathe when you go to bed. Reduce your alcohol consumption and sleep in a peaceful manner.

240.   If you snore, have your nose evaluated for any blockages or architectural problems. You may have a blockage from an injury, or you may have been born with one. A blockage in your nasal passages

does not allow optimal airflow, which causes you to snore. Corrective surgery may be possible to help you stop snoring.

241.   To minimize snoring, try to eat a large breakfast and lunch during the day. This will force you to have a smaller dinner, which is very beneficial towards maintaining a high comfort level when you sleep at night. The more comfortable you are when you rest, the less of a chance for you to snore.

242.   Mouth guards have been known to help people stop snoring. You can get a special mouth guard prescribed to you by your dentist or family doctor. These mouth guards keep your lower jaw from getting too relaxed, and they keep your teeth close together. Have a doctor prescribe a special mouth guard to help you stop snoring.

243.   Dairy products in your diet might be the culprit when someone who sleeps within earshot tells you you have a snoring problem. Staying away from dairy close to bedtime for a week or so, will give you a chance to see if the snoring stops. Dairy can cause mucus to build in the throat of some individuals. When this happens, snoring might be the result. You need not avoid dairy products entirely; simply avoid indulging in them within a few hours of going to bed.

244.   You should not eat or drink dairy products right before you go to sleep. They can cause excess mucus build-up, which in turn causes different breathing, resulting in snoring. There are plenty of other times throughout the day to eat dairy products, so cut out that ice cream before you go to bed.

245.   If you are becoming a nuisance to yourself and someone you love because of snoring, try this tip. Oils, such as peppermint, eucalyptus and menthol have been known to shrink nasal passages, reducing the chances of snoring. Just rub a little around your nostril opening and you should notice a decrease in your snoring.

246.   To help you prevent snoring you should change the position in which you sleep. When you sleep on your back it is said to cause people to snore. So switching positions can reduce or eliminate snoring. Instead of sleeping on your back, try sleeping on your side or stomach to prevent you from snoring.

247.   If you are having trouble dealing with a partner who tends to snore a lot, considering going to sleep before they do so you can at least have a fighting chance of getting some peaceful sleep. If you're a

light sleeper, you may not be able to make this work, but it is worth a try.

248.   It may be worthwhile try a few of the medications or tools available to assist with snoring issues. Many people swear by pills, nasal strips, and sprays. Whichever treatment option you choose to pursue, seek a doctor's advice first in order to discover what will work best for your specific case.

249.   Snoring can be a frustrating thing to deal with, but it may just be an underlying symptom of something larger so make sure you are taking your overall health into consideration. If you are dealing with other health problems, speak with your doctor and find out if your snoring is actually being caused by something more serious such as obesity or even smoking.

250.   The most common reason for snoring in children is enlarged tonsils and adenoids. If you notice that your child has a significant snoring problem, a trip to the pediatrician can tell you for sure if this is the problem. Since snoring can pose health issues in childhood, some doctors recommend the removal of the tonsils and adenoids to eliminate snoring.

251.   One of the most effective ways to stop snoring is to cease alcohol use. When you consume alcohol, the muscles in the back of your throat become too relaxed. This state of relation can increase your chances of snoring. If you really want to drink, only have one or two.

252.   If you suffer from snoring, it is important that you not sleep on your back. This position narrows the airways in your throat, thus, reducing airflow. This lack of air can be a cause of snoring. It is recommended that you sleep on either your right or left side instead.

253.   If snoring has become a nighttime concern, then it is time to give dairy products such as milk, yogurt or cheese a miss before you go to sleep each night. This is because the dairy products can cause mucus to build up near your breathing passages, and this will trigger off snoring.

254.   Try to keep your head elevated when sleeping if you want to prevent snoring. Being in this position allows your muscles and airways to get in just the right amount of air, which lessens the chance that you will snore. Just prop some pillows behind your head or use a thick pillow.

255.   If you are a smoker that snores, your cigarette habit may be a large part of the problem--go ahead and quit. Smoking causes a great deal of damage to the respiratory system and increases the amount of mucus in your airways, which can lead to snoring. Kicking the habit may nip your snoring problems in the bud.

256.   You need to avoid drinking alcohol if you snore. On top of this, you should stay away from antihistamines, sleeping pills and any type of tranquilizer right before you go to bed. Alcohol and sleeping pills are muscle relaxants, and therefore cause the muscles in your throat to collapse. These restrict the passage of air through your system, and cause you to snore.

257.   To deal with snoring and its effects on your relationship, have a clear talk with your partner if he or she is not being very nice to you because of it. Just because you're snoring doesn't mean that your partner should yell at you in the middle of the night. You need to take the step to stop snoring and your partner needs to be understanding, especially if you're doing what you can to remedy the problem.

258.   If you snore, have your nose evaluated for any blockages or architectural problems. You may have a blockage from an injury, or you may have been

born with one. A blockage in your nasal passages does not allow optimal airflow, which causes you to snore. Corrective surgery may be possible to help you stop snoring.

259.   Refrain from sleeping on a mattress that you sink into or is slanted. This will cause your body to be at an angle, which can put tension on your air passages during the night. Try to find a mattress that is parallel to the ground so that you can breathe efficiently without snoring.

260.   One of the ways that you can improve your breathing and eliminate snoring at night is to inhale steam for several minutes before bed. Taking in steam can help to break down your congestion, which can play an integral role in clearing your passages to allow you to sleep efficiently.

261.   If all of your remedies fail, one of the things that you can do is seek professional advice from a doctor. There are many different types of surgeries that you can undergo to increase your air passages so that you can breathe more efficiently at night. Get professional help if your snoring becomes a serious dilemma.

262.   Use a neti pot to reduce your snoring. A neti pot is a specialized device that allows you to purge your

sinuses with warm water. They are available at practically any health food store and can be a tremendous asset in keeping your nasal passages clear so you don't snore.

263.   If you or your partner snores at night, do not sleep isolated from each other. Instead, help prevent snoring from happening as you select plan to deal with it. Sleeping away from each other just strains the relationship and restricts intimacy at night. Keep a healthy relationship, and eliminate snoring from your nightly routine.

264.   To help aid you in not snoring, you should not drink alcohol excessively. Drinking too much alcohol softens the tissues in your throat. When the tissues in your throat get soft, it can make a person snore. Those alcoholic beverages should be kept to a minimum, especially right before bedtime, if you do not want to snore.

265.   If you want to decrease your snoring, then try drinking tea before you go to bed. The best tea to try would be nettle tea which you can purchase from most herbal shops. This type of tea provides a soothing effect and also will reduce inflammations that are caused from allergies related to pollen, dust or dirt. Overall, herbal teas tend to have a calming and relaxing effect.

266.   A good tip for people who wish to eliminate their snoring problem is to stop using any sort of tranquilizer. While it may help you sleep, the muscles in your mouth and throat will be extremely relaxed which actually promotes snoring. Keep them out of your system if you wish to stop snoring.

267.   Most people snore during their deepest sleep while lying on their back. Usually, it is not a problem unless the snoring disturbs their sleeping partner, in which case, they will probably be awakened and be asked to roll on their side. This action is probably the first and oldest cure for snoring.

268.   Allergy and sinus sufferers tend to suffer from snoring. This is because you have too much congestion in your nose, so you are breathing in and out of your mouth when you are sleeping. If you have sinus or allergy issues, getting them properly treated could end your snoring as well.

269.   If you are a snorer, there's a chance that you are unaware of it. Always take into account your partner, as they probably have to deal with it throughout the night, so don't get angry if they complain about your snoring. This is always a good

time to talk to each other and try to figure out a solution.

270.   If you have allergies or another condition that causes congestion, the chances of you snoring are increased. Congested sinuses restrict airflow through the nasal passages, which makes you snore. One suggestion on how to fight this is to use a decongestant before bed in order to have a more peaceful night's sleep.

271.   Reduce or eliminate your alcohol consumption, if you are bothered by snoring. You must also avoid antihistamines, tranquilizers and sleeping pills prior to bedtime. These products cause muscles in your body to relax, so this constricts your airway and can cause you to snore more.

272.   Drinking water is a great way to create a smooth passageway for the air in your body. During the course of the day, drink at least eight glasses of water to maximize hydration. Water will help you to feel refreshed and can aid in breathing freely at night, reducing the chance that you will snore.

273.   Learn to sleep on your side if you do not already. Sleeping on your side helps keep your throat open so that air can move freely in and out. Sleeping on your back makes your throat muscles

slack and prevents good airflow. Interrupted or bad airflow is what causes snoring.

274.   If you snore, have your nose evaluated for any blockages or architectural problems. You may have a blockage from an injury, or you may have been born with one. A blockage in your nasal passages does not allow optimal airflow, which causes you to snore. Corrective surgery may be possible to help you stop snoring.

275.   Always choose a pillow that is firm and elevated several inches off of your bed. This will help tremendously to reduce the strain on your airways so that you do not feel constricted when you breathe. Implementing this technique will result in a much more comfortable night of rest and minimal snoring.

276.   If you are a woman and you have recently started snoring, get your thyroid checked. Sometimes this can be an indication of an underactive thyroid, or hypothyroidism. This hormone imbalance can greatly affect your sleep patterns, because sleep is governed in part by a complex interplay of several different hormones.

277.   Try to not consume overly sugary foods or overly rich foods. Deserts, in particular, aren't a

good choice when you have a tendency to snore. Chocolates, cookies, cakes, and even ice cream are associated with snoring. So too are foods such a pizza, lasagna, and other high-calorie, high-fat, rich foods.

278.   Regularly give your mouth a good work out. Stronger face and jaw muscles can reduce snoring. Purse your lips together tightly and push them as far away from your face as possible. Hold that position for several seconds. Alternately, pull up the edges of your mouth as though you are smiling and hold it there.

279.   Consult your doctor if you have allergies and have started snoring. Seasonal allergies are an often overlooked cause of snoring. A stuffed up nose or clogged sinuses causes you to breathe through your mouth, which can lead to snoring. Your doctor may recommend using a saline spray, humidifier or antihistamine.

280.   Software like Dreamweaver and Adobe Photoshop are highly useful tools for web designers. If you aren't familiar with these programs, investigate them to see how to use them to your advantage.

281.   Exercise regularly in order to reduce or eliminate snoring. You are able to sleep more deeply and soundly if your body has worked hard during the day. All the muscles in your body will benefit from regular exercise, including the ones in your neck. When they are stronger, your throat is less likely to close up while you sleep.

282.   Consider learning to play the musical instrument of choice for the Australian Aborigines, the didgeridoo. This instrument is a long, open-ended tube and can help in your battle against snoring. One end of the didgeridoo is placed against your mouth. Flex the muscles of your throat and blow through your pursed lips to make them rapidly flap. The air that is released resonates into the tube and produces the distinctive sound.

283.   Nasal strips can be very effective in reducing snoring. They stick to your nose and pull up your nostrils, opening them and permitting more air to travel through. Wider nostrils translate to less snoring. But, if you suffer from sleep apnea, you shouldn't use them.

284.   Cut down excess eating and alcohol consumption for a few hours before bed, to decrease your snoring chances. Alcohol and eating heavy meals tend to relax the throat muscles. When

your throat muscles are too relax, snoring can occur.

285.   Smoking causes your throat to swell, which in turn causes you to snore at night. One good way to prevent snoring is to stop smoking now. Try a smoking cessation class, over-the-counter nicotine patches or a prescription medication from your doctor. You will not only improve your health and prevent lung cancer, but you will sleep better at night.

286.   Avoid drinking alcohol within 5 hours of bedtime. Alcohol, along with other sedative drugs, causes the muscles at the back of the throat to relax. When these muscles relax, you are more apt to snore. Stay away from those nightcaps--you may actually sleep more soundly if you do not drink before bed.

287.   The strange thing is that taking sleeping pills can result in snoring. Skip them, and you will be less likely to snore. The main effect of sleeping pills is to relax every one of your muscles. The muscles in your nasal passages will also relax, which makes the passages smaller. The result is the snoring sound as the air moves through these restricted air ways.

288.   In order to cut back on snoring, turn over and sleep on your side, not on your back. If you sleep on your back, especially with only one or two pillows, mucus can gather in your nasal passages. Sleeping on your side will keep the mucus out of the passages, and you won't have a blockage that will cause snoring.

289.   To reduce snoring, keep your airways open. A clogged nose, or one that is otherwise constricted, may contribute to snoring. Use neti pots, steam showers, eucalyptus rubs and humidifiers to keep your nose clear when you are ill. Nasal strips can also help you because they actually lift your nose open, allowing air to enter.

290.   A way to avoid the snoring that comes with extremely deep sleep is to develop and keep a steady sleep routine. If your body is accustomed to resting at a certain time, that sleep will be calmer, and you'll snore less. Getting a regular 8 hours a night, at the same time each night, will make sleeping more beneficial (and quieter for those around you).

291.   Try to keep your head elevated when sleeping if you want to prevent snoring. Being in this position allows your muscles and airways to get in just the right amount of air, which lessens the chance that

you will snore. Just prop some pillows behind your head or use a thick pillow.

292.   Do not consume dairy before going to bed. Dairy products may cause a build up of mucus in your respiratory system and this build up causes snoring. Do not eat ice cream, drink milk or consume any other dairy products before bed and this can help you avoid snoring.

293.   Consider using a chin strap to keep your snoring under control. Chin straps keep your mouth closed so it is difficult to snore. These devices are available in a wide variety of styles. Many are elastic and simply fit over your head. Others are fitted with Velcro so they can be custom adjusted to fit your head.

294.   There are several methods to help you stop snoring by building throat muscles. One of these requires you to stand in front of the mirror and open your mouth. Work the muscle in the rear of your throat. If you're contracting that muscle correctly, you'll see the uvula bobbing up and down -- and you'll stop snoring.

295.   Side sleeping is a great way to prevent snoring. If you sleep on your back, the chance of you snoring is greater. If you sleep on your stomach,

you may cause undue stress to your neck. Refraining from sleeping on your back and instead opting for your side will be more ideal for you.

296.   Sleep in an elevated position to help reduce your snoring. Sleeping in a horizontal position can put more pressure on your airway causing it to close. By elevating your whole upper body and not just your head, you can relieve this extra pressure. Try propping your whole torso up on pillows or putting some blocks beneath your bedposts at the head of your bed.

297.   As with so many other health issues, obesity definitely increases the occurrences of snoring. A recent increase in snoring could easily be the result of a recent increase in weight. Even if losing that weight does not completely solve your snoring problem, you can only gain from getting more fit.

298.   If you suffer from allergies, and you snore, seek the advice of your doctor. There may be medicine or shots you can take to reduce your allergies. Reducing the symptoms of allergies like nasal stuffiness, can help reduce snoring. Make sure you let your doctor know about the snoring, so that you don't end up with a medicine that relaxes your throat muscles.

299.   To reduce snoring, train yourself to breathe through your nose. There are snoring strips on the market that adhere across the bridge of the nose. They open the nasal passages to encourage nasal breathing. These can be used in conjunction with chin straps to prevent the mouth from opening while you sleep.

300.   Losing weight is a good step to take in order to stop snoring at night while you are asleep. Extra weight restricts breathing, especially extra weight around the neck. Maintain a balanced diet, exercise, and lose a few pounds to help remedy your breathing and snoring issues.

301.   If you have a snoring problem, avoid sleeping on your back. This position makes snoring more likely because of the way the soft palate and base of the tongue rest at the back of your mouth. Instead, sleep on your side. You are less likely to snore in this position and your quality of sleep will likely improve.

302.   Believe it or not, you can effectively beat snoring by repeating your vowels a few times a day. What this does is move around muscles in your throat and face and when these muscles get stronger, your chances of snoring are slim to none. You can do this three times a day.

303.   If you wish to prevent snoring, you should ensure that your nasal passages are open. If your nose is clogged or swollen, you are more likely to snore. If you catch a cold try and unclog your nose by using vapor rubs, humidifiers, or steam showers. You may want to consider using nasal strips as a means to opening up your nasal passageway, which allows you to breath easier.

304.   Drinking alcohol too close to bedtime can result in snoring. This happens because alcohol tends to relax the throat muscles, which leads to tightened airways. As a result, snoring is more likely to occur. The best way to avoid snoring due to alcohol consumption is to stop drinking spirits at least 5 to 6 hours before bedtime.

305.   To limit your level of snoring during the night, refrain from smoking altogether. Smoking can constrict your airways, which can make it much harder for you to breathe at night. This will not only help you to reduce the intensity of your snoring but make you feel better as the night wears on.

306.   One of the best ways to eliminate snoring during the night is to cut down on your intake of alcohol during the day. Alcohol tends to tighten your airways, which will make it much harder to

breathe when you go to bed. Reduce your alcohol consumption and sleep in a peaceful manner.

307.   Ready to stop snoring? There are some throat exercises you can do to keep your throat muscles stronger. One thing you can do is repeat the five vowels out loud, consistently, for three minutes consecutively, several times a day. Building your throat muscles will reduce your instances of snoring.

308.   Treat your allergies if you have a tendency to snore at night. If you are congested or your respiratory system is irritated, you will be more likely to snore when you go to sleep. Use a decongestant or an antihistamine to treat your allergies, and keep your airway clear at night.

309.   Lose as much excess weight as possible. Extra weight does not just show up in your thighs, it can make your throat narrower. This can cause snoring and sleep apnea. Even a 10 pound loss can help open up the passageway in your throat. The more wide open it is, the better you will sleep.

310.   Humidify the air in your bedroom if you have a snoring problem. When you breathe in dry air all night as you sleep, your throat and nasal membranes dry out. This leads to swelling and

congestion that narrows your airways. That constriction makes it difficult to get enough air and causes you to snore.

311.   Use nasal strips at night before you go to sleep. When you apply a strip to your nose, it will open both of your nostrils to let in more air. When the nasal passage is constricted, it can exacerbate the tendency to snore. Using nasal strips will result in a reduction in snoring.

312.   Make your bedroom as allergy-proof as you can. If you suffer from allergies, it is important that you try to prevent congestion due to allergic reactions from affecting your sleep. Congestion during sleep leads to snoring. Remove as many of your allergy triggers as possible from your bedroom in order to give yourself the best chance of enjoying a peaceful night's rest.

313.   Don't eat a large meal right before going to bed for the night. Doing so will cause your full stomach to push up on your diaphragm. This can obstruct your airways, limit your breathing and keep you from being able to take full, deep breaths which leads to snoring.

314.   Do you snore? Give singing a try. Singing is a natural form of exercise for the muscles in the

throat and soft palate. Since snoring is sometimes caused by lax muscles in these areas, strengthening them can help. So go ahead and belt out your favorite tune every day. Your partner might just sleep better because they no longer have to listen to you snore!

315.   In order to eliminate your snoring, you may need to ask your doctor or dentist about getting a mouth guard. These things can hold your teeth together and prevent your lower jaw muscles from being too loose when you are sleeping. This method is one of the most effective ones for eliminating snoring.

316.   If you snore and you are a smoker, then you should consider quitting smoking. Smoking causes damage to your respiratory system, which causes you to snore louder. Therefore, you need to quit smoking so that you can not only achieve better health, but you can also quit your annoying snoring at night.

317.   There are many different remedies on the market that may help reduce or eliminate snoring. On the market, you'll find nasal strips, pills and sprays that have worked for many snorers. Regardless of what you try, always consult a

physician first, so they can make a recommendation about what the best option is for your problem.

318.   If you regularly use cigarettes and other tobacco products, you probably also snore. The ingredients in these products dries out the mucosal membranes in your nose, mouth and airway, which leads to difficulty breathing and loud snoring. If at all possible, do not smoke cigarettes within five hours of your bedtime as the smoke will cause your airway to become inflamed.

319.   Facial exercises do more than just tone and trim your jawline; actually, by regularly completing these exercises, you may also strengthen the muscles of your mouth and neck. As a result, you will be less prone to loud and disruptive snoring throughout the night. Now THAT, is really something to smile about!

320.   Don't drink alcoholic beverages before going to bed. The very reason you might be tempted to have a nighttime drink, the fact that you want to relax, can cause you to snore. When your muscles relax because of the alcohol, so do your air passages. As your air passages become restricted, you snore.

321.   Losing weight should help you reduce your snoring. Excess fat in your neck can increase

pressure in your throat, which can cause narrowing of your airways. This causes your airways to partially collapse during the night. By losing only a few pound, you can significantly decrease your snoring.

322.   Use nasal strips at night before you go to sleep. When you apply a strip to your nose, it will open both of your nostrils to let in more air. When the nasal passage is constricted, it can exacerbate the tendency to snore. Using nasal strips will result in a reduction in snoring.

323.   You can often reduce snoring using a simple tennis ball. Prior to going to bed, attach the ball to your nightwear. Each time you roll over onto your back, the ball will prompt you to switch back to your side. If you sleep on your side, you will notice a significant reduction in your snoring.

324.   If you have a problem with snoring, sinus infections may be a cause for you to look into. Sinus infection can block airways, making it hard to breathe. This can cause the passages to create a vacuum which can lead to snoring. Nasal infection can cause snoring in the same way.

325.   Snoring can be a problem if you are used to sleeping on your back. This position can cause the tissues in the throat to become lax which can in

turn block your airway, causing snoring. Try to sleep in a different position, such as on your side to eliminate this problem.

326.   Wearing nasal strips while you are sleeping ensures a continuous opening of your nasal air passages, which can help alleviate much of your snoring. Try wearing nasal strips at night while you are sleeping, and see how they work for you. Using them in conjunction with other tips has been known to significantly reduce how much a person snores.

327.   People with asthma have an increased chance of snoring regularly at night. If you have asthma, you should consult your doctor to see what you can do about snoring prevention. Whatever you are required to do for your asthma in general is also important, as this keeps you breathing regularly, reducing how often you snore.

328.   When dealing with a partner that snores, it can be rather annoying. However, you must remember that he or she is not doing it to you on purpose. Search for snoring remedies, so that you both can get some sleep at night.

329.   Exercise regularly in order to reduce or eliminate snoring. You are able to sleep more deeply and

soundly if your body has worked hard during the day. All the muscles in your body will benefit from regular exercise, including the ones in your neck. When they are stronger, your throat is less likely to close up while you sleep.

330.   Sleeping pills or alcohol can actually help to reduce your snoring. This can work because of the inherent ability of these chemicals to relax your body, including throat muscles. Muscles that are overactive can contribute to snoring. Use with caution, as alcohol and sleeping pills can increase the risk of sleep apnea.

331.   One problem that common snorers ignore is the effects it has on one's relationship with a spouse or partner. Snoring can cause anger, frustration, and ultimately, separate sleeping arrangements. Since snoring is bad for a relationship, it's important to seek treatment early!

332.   Chronic snorers who also have sleep apnea should consult their doctor about the possibility of a cpap machine. This device has a mask you wear at night while sleeping which delivers oxygen and air to keep your passages open which will prevent snoring. It is recommended for people with sever snoring and apnea problems.

333.   Many people suffer from snoring that is caused by nasal congestion or allergies. If this is the case, then trying an allergy medicine or spray a few hours before you go to sleep may be the answer. This will give it time to start working at clearing your passages by the time you go to bed.

334.   A good tip for people who wish to eliminate their snoring problem is to stop using any sort of tranquilizer. While it may help you sleep, the muscles in your mouth and throat will be extremely relaxed which actually promotes snoring. Keep them out of your system if you wish to stop snoring.

9 781978 475861